Hepatic steatosis

Understand the role of diet and lifestyle in managing fatty liver disease

Dr Walt wade

Contents

Chapter1

introduction to fatty liver disease

Fatty liver disease, also known as hepatic steatosis, is a condition in which excessive fat accumulates in the liver, leading to inflammation and damage to the liver cells. This disease is becoming increasingly common, with an estimated 100 million people in the United States alone affected by it. It is a serious health concern, as it can lead to complications such as cirrhosis, liver failure, and even liver cancer. In this article, we will delve into what fatty liver disease is, its causes, symptoms, and treatment options. Fatty liver disease can be categorized into two main types: non-alcoholic fatty liver disease (NAFLD) and alcoholic fatty liver disease (AFLD).

NAFLD is the more common type and is not caused by excessive alcohol consumption. It is often associated with other health conditions such as obesity, diabetes, and high cholesterol. AFLD, on the other hand, is a result of excessive alcohol consumption and is typically seen in heavy drinkers. The main cause of fatty liver disease is the build-up of fat in the liver cells, which can be caused by various factors. One common cause of NAFLD is an unhealthy lifestyle, characterized by a diet high in processed and fatty foods, lack of exercise, and excessive alcohol consumption. These habits lead to the deposition of fat in the liver, which can eventually lead to inflammation and damage. Another underlying cause of fatty liver disease is insulin resistance. Insulin is a hormone that helps regulate the body's blood sugar levels. When the body becomes resistant to insulin, it can result in elevated levels of insulin in the blood, which can lead to the accumulation of fat in the liver. This condition is commonly seen in people with obesity and type 2 diabetes. Genetics may also play a role in the development of fatty liver disease. Certain genes can make individuals more susceptible to this condition. Studies have shown that having a family history of NAFLD increases the risk of developing the disease. Fatty liver disease often does not show any symptoms in its early stages. However, as the disease progresses, symptoms may start to appear. Some of the common signs and symptoms of fatty liver disease include fatigue, pain in the upper right side of the abdomen, swelling in the stomach, and jaundice (yellowing of the skin and eyes). If left untreated, fatty liver disease can lead to more severe symptoms such as confusion, bleeding disorders, and even liver failure. If you are experiencing any of these symptoms, it is important to consult with a healthcare professional. A diagnosis of fatty liver disease is typically confirmed through blood tests, imaging tests such as ultrasound or MRI, and a liver biopsy. Treatment for fatty liver disease depends on its underlying cause and severity. For NAFLD, lifestyle modifications are key to managing the disease. This includes a healthy diet, regular exercise, and avoiding alcohol consumption. In some cases, medications may be prescribed to control high cholesterol or insulin resistance. Weight loss has also been shown to significantly improve fatty liver disease. For those with AFLD, the most crucial step to treatment is to stop consuming alcohol. This may be a difficult process for heavy drinkers and may require medical interventions and support. In some cases, fatty liver disease may progress to a more severe stage, known as non-alcoholic steatohepatitis (NASH). This is characterized by inflammation and damage to the liver cells, which can eventually lead to cirrhosis and liver failure. In such cases, more intensive treatment, such as liver transplantation, may be required. Prevention is the best approach to managing fatty liver disease. Maintaining a healthy weight, having a balanced diet, and limiting alcohol consumption are key to preventing the disease. Regular exercise is also important as it helps reduce insulin resistance and improve overall liver function. In conclusion, fatty liver disease is a common and serious condition that can have severe consequences if left untreated. It is essential to understand its causes, symptoms, and available treatment options. Making lifestyle modifications and seeking medical advice can help manage the disease and prevent it from progressing to more severe stages. With the right measures, fatty liver disease can be effectively managed, leading to a healthier liver and an improved quality of life.

Chapter2

The Role of Diet and Lifestyle in Managing Fatty Liver Disease"

The liver is a vital organ responsible for a variety of functions, including filtering toxins from the blood, producing bile for digestion, and storing glycogen for energy. When the liver is overwhelmed with excess fat, it becomes less efficient in performing its duties, which can lead to various health complications and even progress to more severe conditions, such as liver fibrosis, cirrhosis, and liver cancer. Therefore, managing fatty liver disease is crucial to prevent further damage and improve overall health. One of the main factors contributing to fatty liver disease is an unhealthy diet. Consuming a high amount of unhealthy fats, such as saturated and trans fats, can lead to a buildup of fat in the liver cells. These fats are commonly found in processed and fried foods, red meat, and high-fat dairy products. A diet high in simple carbohydrates, such as sugary drinks and snacks, can also promote the development of fatty liver disease. These simple carbs are converted into fat in the liver, adding to the already existing fat accumulation. On the other hand, a healthy diet can play a significant role in managing and even reversing fatty liver disease. A Mediterranean-style diet, which includes plenty of fruits, vegetables, whole grains, lean protein, and healthy fats, has been shown to be beneficial in reducing liver fat and improving liver function. This type of diet is rich in antioxidants, which can help reduce inflammation in the liver and prevent further damage. Additionally, a Mediterranean diet is lower in simple carbs and unhealthy fats, making it a suitable choice for those with fatty liver disease. In addition to a healthy diet, maintaining a healthy weight is crucial in managing fatty liver disease. Obesity is a significant risk factor for the development and progression of NAFLD. People with a body mass index (BMI) of 30 or higher are at a higher risk of developing fatty liver disease. Losing weight can help reduce the amount of fat in the liver and improve liver function. Experts recommend aiming for a gradual weight loss of 1-2 pounds per week by making healthier food choices and incorporating regular physical activity into one's routine. Regular exercise is not only beneficial for weight loss but also directly affects liver health. Physical activity can help reduce liver fat, improve insulin sensitivity, and lower inflammation in the body. Engaging in moderate-intensity exercise, such as brisk walking, for at least 30 minutes a day, five days a week, is recommended for individuals with fatty liver disease. Strength training exercises can also be beneficial in reducing liver fat and improving overall health. Apart from diet and exercise, certain lifestyle changes can also help manage fatty liver disease. Limiting or avoiding alcohol consumption is essential for those with NAFLD. Alcohol is toxic to liver cells and can worsen liver damage in people with fatty liver disease. Experts recommend limiting alcohol intake to one drink per day for women and two drinks per day for men. Quitting smoking is also essential, as smoking can contribute to liver damage and worsen the condition of people with fatty liver disease. Another crucial aspect of managing fatty liver disease is monitoring and managing other health conditions. People with NAFLD are at a higher risk of developing other health problems, such as type 2 diabetes, high blood pressure, and high cholesterol levels. Therefore, it is essential to monitor and manage these conditions to prevent further damage to the liver and overall health. A well-balanced diet, regular exercise, and medication, if necessary, can help control these health issues and improve liver function. In addition to these lifestyle changes, there are also specific dietary supplements that have been shown to have a positive impact on fatty liver disease. Supplements such as vitamin E, omega-3 fatty acids, and milk thistle have been studied for their potential to reduce liver fat and improve liver function in people with NAFLD. However, it is essential to consult with a healthcare professional before starting any supplements, as they may interact with other medications or have potential side effects.

Chapter3

"The Link between Obesity and Fatty Liver Disease

Obesity and fatty liver disease, also known as non-alcoholic fatty liver disease (NAFLD), are two major health issues that are closely linked to one another. In fact, obesity is one of the leading risk factors for developing fatty liver disease. In this essay, we will explore the link between these two conditions, their impact on health, and ways to prevent and treat them. Firstly, it is important to understand what obesity and fatty liver disease are. Obesity refers to an excessive accumulation of body fat, usually caused by consuming more calories than one burns through physical activity. It is commonly measured by body mass index (BMI) which is calculated by dividing one's weight (in kilograms) by their height squared (in meters). A BMI of 30 or higher is considered obese. On the other hand, fatty liver disease is a condition where excess fat builds up in the liver, leading to inflammation and liver damage. It is estimated that about 20-30% of the global population has fatty liver disease, making it a widespread health concern. So how are these two conditions related? The main link between obesity and fatty liver disease is the presence of excess fat in the body. In obese individuals, the excess fat is mainly stored in adipose tissue, but when the body's fat storage capacity is reached, the fat starts to accumulate in other organs, including the liver. This leads to the development of fatty liver disease. In some cases, fatty liver disease can also lead to obesity, creating a vicious cycle where both conditions exacerbate each other. The impact of obesity and fatty liver disease on health is significant. Obesity increases the risk of developing a range of health problems, including diabetes, heart disease, stroke, and certain types of cancer. Fatty liver disease, if left untreated, can progress to a more serious condition called non-alcoholic steatohepatitis (NASH), which can lead to liver fibrosis, cirrhosis, and even liver failure. Additionally, both obesity and fatty liver disease are associated with increased inflammation in the body, which can further contribute to the development of chronic diseases. Fortunately, both obesity and fatty liver disease can be prevented and treated. The most effective prevention strategy is maintaining a healthy lifestyle. This includes following a balanced diet, engaging in regular physical activity, and managing stress levels. In terms of diet, it is important to limit the intake of processed and high-fat foods and opt for a diet rich in fruits, vegetables, whole grains, and lean proteins. Regular exercise, at least 30 minutes a day, can also help not only with weight management but also with improving liver health. Furthermore, for individuals who are already obese or have fatty liver disease, weight loss is a crucial step in managing and improving their condition. Studies have shown that even a modest weight loss of 5-10% can significantly decrease the amount of fat in the liver and improve liver function. This can be achieved through a combination of a healthy diet and exercise, as well as seeking guidance from healthcare professionals. In addition, there are certain medications that can help treat fatty liver disease, particularly if weight loss alone is not enough. These medications work by reducing the amount of fat accumulated in the liver and improving its function. However, these medications should only be taken under the supervision of a doctor. In some cases, fatty liver disease can progress to more severe liver conditions, such as NASH or cirrhosis.

In these cases, more advanced treatments such as liver transplantation may be necessary. However, these treatments can be avoided by managing and treating obesity and fatty liver disease in the early stages.

Chapter4

Breaking Down the Stages and Progression of Fatty Liver Disease"

Stage 1: Simple fatty liver The first stage of fatty liver disease is known as simple fatty liver, or hepatic steatosis. In this stage, there is an abnormal accumulation of fat in the liver cells, without any inflammation or damage. Often, this stage does not produce any noticeable symptoms, and the condition can only be diagnosed through imaging tests or a liver biopsy. Simple fatty liver can be caused by factors such as excessive alcohol consumption, obesity, and high-fat diet. Stage 2: Non-alcoholic steatohepatitis (NASH) If the accumulation of fat in the liver is accompanied by inflammation and liver cell damage, the condition progresses to non-alcoholic steatohepatitis (NASH). In this stage, the liver becomes swollen and tender, and there may be scarring or fibrosis. The symptoms of NASH may include fatigue, weakness, and abdominal discomfort. If NASH is diagnosed early, it can be reversed with lifestyle changes such as weight loss, regular exercise, and a healthy diet. However, if left untreated, it can progress to more severe stages of fatty liver disease. Stage 3: Fibrosis In the third stage, the inflammation and damage in the liver lead to the formation of scar tissue, also known as fibrosis. As the disease progresses, the fibrotic tissue can block the flow of blood and impair liver function. At this stage, the symptoms become more pronounced, and liver function tests may show abnormal results. The liver can still recover at this stage with proper lifestyle changes and medical treatment, but the risk of developing cirrhosis increases. Stage 4: Cirrhosis Cirrhosis is the most advanced stage of fatty liver disease, in which the liver becomes severely scarred and cannot function properly. The scarring leads to irreversible damage, and the liver is unable to perform its vital functions, such as filtering toxins from the blood and producing important proteins. Symptoms of cirrhosis may include jaundice, fluid buildup in the abdomen, and mental confusion. At this stage, the complications of fatty liver disease become life-threatening, and a liver transplant may be the only viable treatment option. Progression of fatty liver disease The progression of fatty liver disease can vary from person to person, depending on various factors such as the underlying cause and individual risk factors. In some cases, the disease may not progress beyond the first stage, and the liver may be able to heal itself with lifestyle changes. However, in other cases, it can progress rapidly, leading to severe complications. Studies have shown that certain risk factors can contribute to the progression of fatty liver disease. These include a high intake of sugar and saturated fat, lack of physical activity, and genetics. Patients with obesity, type 2 diabetes, and metabolic syndrome are also at a higher risk of developing severe fatty liver disease. Importance of early detection and management Early detection of fatty liver disease is crucial in preventing its progression to more advanced stages. Due to the lack of noticeable symptoms in the early stages, the disease often goes undiagnosed and untreated, leading to serious complications in the later stages. Therefore, routine check-ups, especially for individuals with risk factors, are essential for early detection. Management of fatty liver disease aims to slow down or reverse the progression of the disease. In the early stages, lifestyle changes such as weight loss, regular exercise, and a healthy diet have been found to be effective in treating fatty liver disease. In more advanced stages, medical treatment may be necessary, which can include medications to reduce inflammation and control blood sugar and cholesterol levels.

"The Role of Exercise in Preventing and Managing Fatty Liver Disease

Exercise has been shown to have numerous benefits for overall health and well-being, and its role in preventing and managing fatty liver disease is no exception. Let's explore the various ways in which exercise can help prevent and manage this condition. 1. Helps with weight management Obesity is one of the key risk factors for fatty liver disease. When we exercise, we burn calories and use up excess fat for energy. This helps to reduce the amount of fat stored in the liver and other parts of the body. In fact, a study published in the journal Hepatology found that aerobic exercise, such as cycling or running, for 60 minutes three times a week for eight weeks, led to a significant reduction in liver fat in people with fatty liver disease. Exercise also helps to increase muscle mass and metabolism, which can further aid in weight management. As we build muscle, our body's resting metabolic rate increases, meaning we burn more calories even when we are at rest. This can help in preventing the development of fatty liver disease in the first place. 2. Improves insulin sensitivity Insulin resistance is a major contributing factor to the development of fatty liver disease. When our cells become resistant to insulin, the body is unable to effectively use glucose for energy, leading to an increase in blood sugar levels. The liver then converts this excess glucose into fat, which can accumulate in the liver. Regular exercise has been shown to improve insulin sensitivity, meaning our cells become more responsive to insulin. This helps to regulate blood sugar levels and reduce fat buildup in the liver. A study conducted at the University of Alabama at Birmingham found that combining aerobic exercise with resistance training for 16 weeks significantly improved insulin sensitivity in individuals with fatty liver disease. 3. Lowers cholesterol and triglyceride levels Elevated levels of cholesterol and triglycerides in the blood are linked to the development of fatty liver disease. Exercise has been shown to have a significant impact on reducing these levels. A study published in the Journal of Hepatology found that 30 minutes of moderate-intensity exercise five times a week for eight weeks led to a significant reduction in both cholesterol and triglyceride levels in individuals with fatty liver disease. Regular exercise can also help to increase the levels of "good" HDL cholesterol in the blood, which helps to remove excess cholesterol from the body. This can further aid in the prevention and management of fatty liver disease. 4.

Reduces inflammation Inflammation is a key component of fatty liver disease and can lead to further damage to the liver. Exercise has been found to have anti-inflammatory effects, which can be beneficial for individuals with fatty liver disease. Studies have shown that regular exercise can reduce the levels of inflammatory markers in the body, leading to a decrease in liver inflammation and improvement in liver function. 5. Increases liver blood flow and oxygen delivery Exercise increases heart rate and blood flow to various parts of the body, including the liver. This increased blood flow and oxygen delivery can help to improve liver function and support the removal of toxins from the body. Additionally, exercise has been found to improve liver blood flow and oxygen delivery even in individuals with cirrhosis, a more advanced form of fatty liver disease. 6. Manages stress and improves mental health Living with a chronic condition like fatty liver disease can be stressful and can take a toll on one's mental health. Exercise has been proven to have positive effects on mental health by reducing stress, anxiety, and depression. It triggers the release of endorphins, also known as the "feel-good" hormones, which can improve mood and overall well-being. Incorporating regular exercise into one's routine can help to alleviate the mental and emotional toll of living with fatty liver disease.

The end